Cancer in My Family

An easy-to-read guide
to better health
for all ages

Co-written by mother/daughter team

Demetra Tsavaris-Lecourezos
Katerina Lecourezos (narrator)

Illustrations by

Leslie Cronkhite Armstrong

First edition 2019
Published in the USA by *thewordverve inc.*
(www.thewordverve.com)

Hardback ISBN: 978-1-948225-77-9
Library of Congress Control Number: 2019916698

~~~~~

Cancer in My Family

Books with Verve by thewordverve inc.

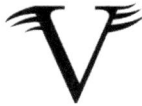

V

Cover Art by Leslie Cronkhite Armstrong
www.scbwi.org/members-public/leslie-armstrong

Cover and Interior Design by Robin Krauss
www.bookformatters.com

As unfortunate as life may seem, we must remember that there is always someone else who is struggling through something so much worse. Always. We feel we are truly blessed . . . blessed to have a strong, willing, and available family; blessed to have dedicated friends; and blessed to have one another.

"Let food be thy medicine, and medicine be thy food."
— Hippocrates, the father of modern medicine

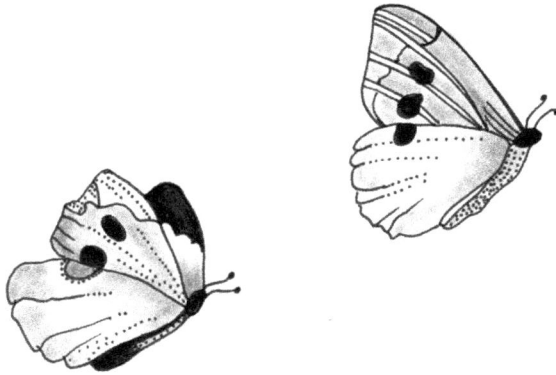

"Learn to enjoy every minute of your life. Be happy now. Don't wait for something outside of yourself to make you happy in the future. Think how really precious is the time you have to spend, whether it's at work or with your family. Every minute should be enjoyed and savored."
— Earl Nightingale

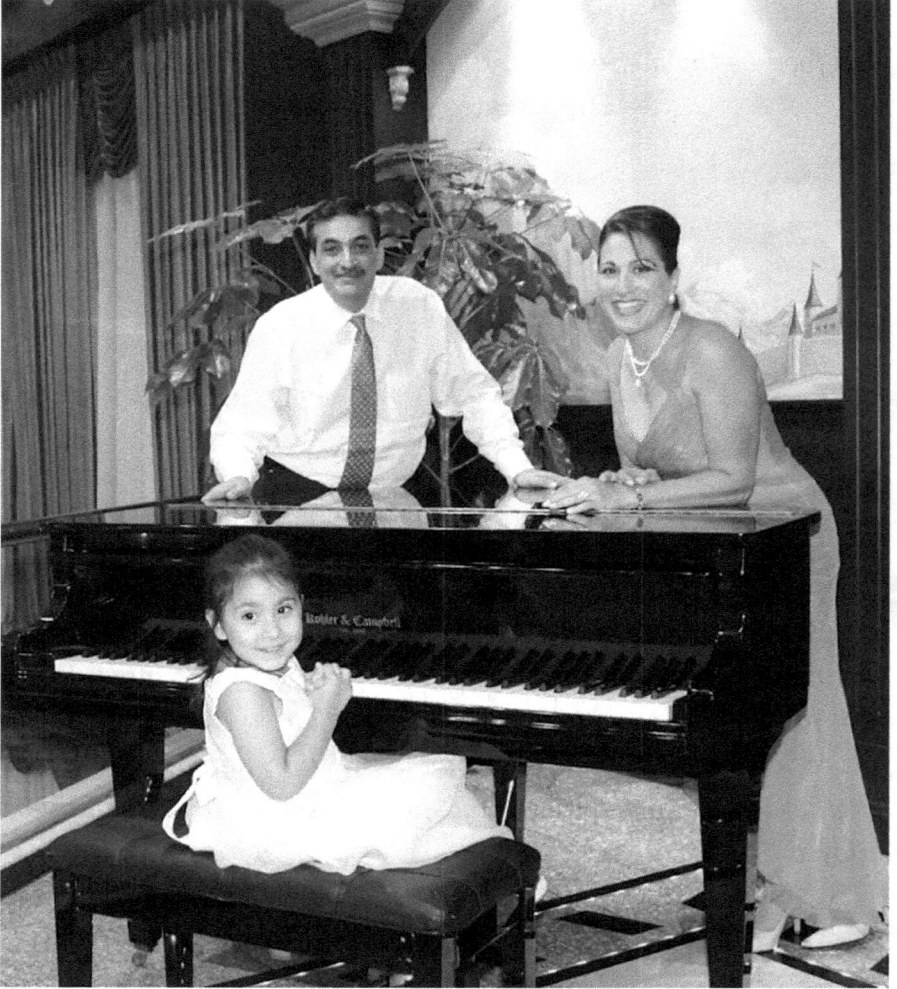

Demetra, Gus and Katerina back in the day.
(Photo credit: Maria Tolios Photography)

Introduction

Even though I am still young, in my early teens, I have quite a story to share about cancer and the impact it has had on my beloved family.

My mom and dad were high school sweethearts. Twenty-one years after going to prom together, they bumped into each other on a street in Manhattan. A year later, they got engaged. A year after that, they got married. And the next year, I was born!

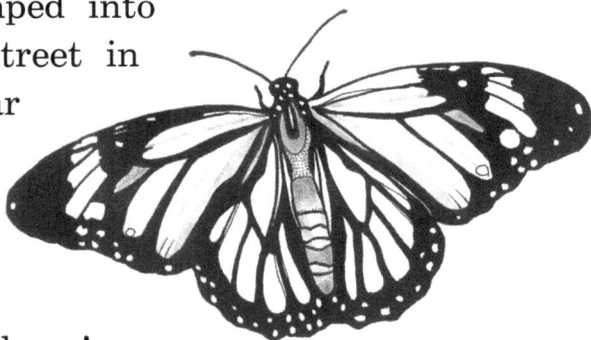

My parents had been married just five years when my dad passed away from pancreatic cancer. I was four years old at the time. I still remember so much about him, though. Mom and I talk about him every single day, and we have loads of pictures of him all over the house.

The three things that I love to talk about most: our trip to Disney when I was four, when he helped me blow out my candles on my third birthday cake, and when he and mom teased one another in the hospital on his last Halloween. Dad was George Clooney for the day, and Mom was Jasmine from Aladdin. I love telling that story!

Now, if that wasn't bad enough, at the same time my dad was sick, my mom's mom was diagnosed with leukemia, another type of cancer. Believe it or not, my Yiayia Eva was really a very fortunate woman. She lived to be eighty-five years old, even though she'd suffered from four different kinds of cancer throughout her life: skin, thyroid, and colon cancer, and finally the leukemia. I say she was fortunate because her doctors always found her cancer early enough that she didn't need chemo or radiation. They were able to operate and remove all the cancer each time, except for the leukemia, which is cancer in the blood. They gave her blood transfusions, but she had a tough time. She was so tired and really just wanted God to take her. What I remember most about Yiayia Eva is that she would sit in her driveway everyday just waiting for me to arrive. She always had this huge smile and would open her arms for me to run to her. She would holler, "My koukla!" which means "doll" in Greek.

After my dad and Yiayia Eva passed away, my mom and I moved to Florida to start a new life. It was going well. My mom had opened her own business. I was in school making new friends, and we were very involved with our church and the community. My mom was having a lot of pain in her leg, and it was really swollen all the time. She figured it was from climbing ladders and working on her knees decorating for events. She finally went to her orthopedic doctor, had an x-ray and MRI done. Guess what? He told her she needed to get to an oncologist—that's a doctor for cancer.

My mom was also diagnosed with a cancer called lymphoma. Then, believe it or not, while we were creating this book, Mom had surgery to remove yet another type of cancer, squamous cell carcinoma, which is a form of skin cancer. You just never know what tomorrow brings.

— Katerina

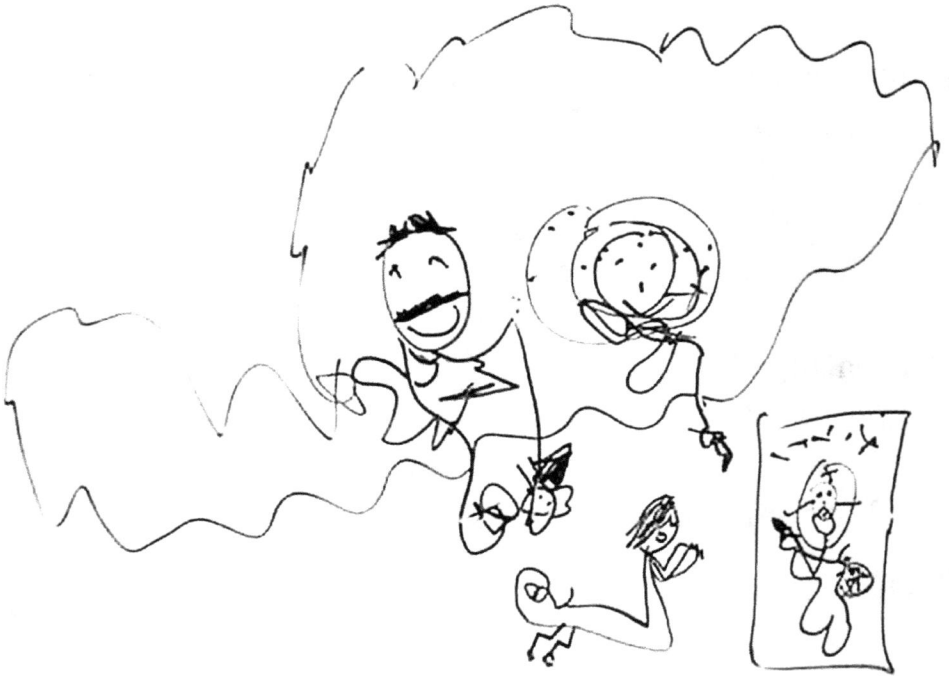

I drew this when I was five years old. My dad (the one with the mustache) is up in heaven, next to Jesus (wearing His halo). My dad is releasing butterflies down to me. That's me kneeling and praying in front of an icon of Jesus.

— Katerina

CHAPTER 1

So many types of cancer

I was amazed to discover how many different types of cancer there are—too numerous to list here, but they can cause different symptoms, if any at all. There are also different ways to treat the cancers.

Pancreatic cancer is one which is very difficult to treat. Once you show any symptoms, it is often too late for the doctors to help the patient. That is the type of cancer my dad had.

His doctors had explained to my mom that there is a direct connection between smoking those nasty cigarettes and pancreatic cancer. Even though my dad never smoked in front of me, he was a very heavy smoker and had been since his teenage years. When my mom told me that, I was shocked. I'd never seen him smoke.

I now understand smoking doesn't always cause cancer, but it certainly increases the risk. Maybe, just maybe, if he hadn't started smoking so young, he would still be with me today.

I was in the room when my mom was told to see an oncologist, but I didn't know that word and didn't

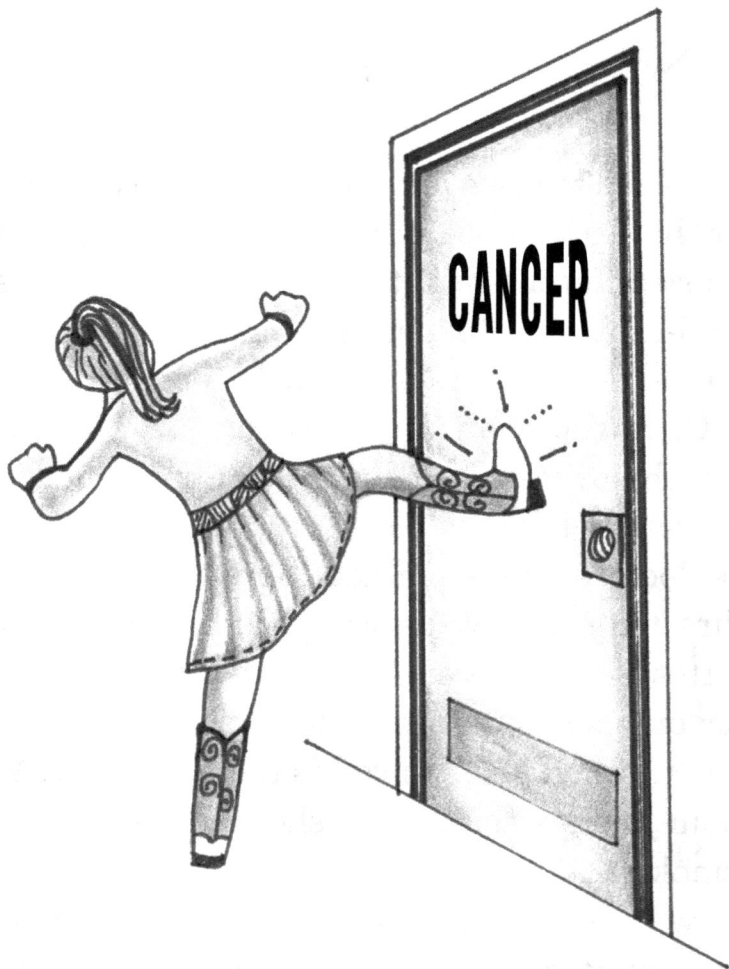

Kicking the door down on cancer.

understand what was happening. She is in remission now. Apparently, five years is the magic number to be able to say "cancer free." We are anxiously waiting for that day to celebrate! One day at a time . . .

With each day that goes by, I learn more and more about my mom's lymphoma, like there are apparently several different types of lymphomas. My mom has what is called "B-cell" or "soft-cell" lymphoma in the soft cell tissues surrounding her right knee. The cancer had spread to her femur bone—the thigh bone—which is why she had so much pain when she walked. The cancer had damaged the muscle. It had also spread to the lymph nodes in her groin. But the doctors told us it is treatable. In fact, they were right, as my mom has improved after undergoing both chemotherapy and then radiation.

Squamous carcinoma is a very common form of skin cancer and is usually caused by UV rays from the sun. Mom is really not a sun-worshipper. In her case, based on where it is located, the squamous was probably caused by the radiation she had received to zap the cancer in her groin.

Even though Mom goes every six months for her PT scan and MRI, the skin cancer they eventually found hadn't shown up on those scans—the doctors said that was typical. This just goes to show how important it is to be vigilant and diligent with our bodies.

Like all cancer patients, my mom asked many questions, such as:

"Why did I get cancer? I don't smoke, do drugs, or even drink alcohol. How could this happen?"

"Is lymphoma hereditary?" (My mom is so concerned about what my future has in store for me as it relates to my health.)

Her biggest question was: "I've got cancer! Now what?"

Of course, I was thinking the same thing.

My mom didn't tell me right away. She waited until she completed her first round of treatments and told me that very night. She wanted me to see that she was okay. I remember crying, and I asked her if she was going to die, just like Dad and Yiayia Eva did. But she explained to me that lymphoma is a very different type of cancer from pancreatic cancer. She told me that she had chemotherapy that day, and said, "Look at me. I am fine." She also explained what medicines the doctors were giving her and some of the side effects to expect, such as losing her hair, being very tired, vision changes, and vomiting.

We discussed what types of tests they would be doing to kick that cancer out the door. The doctors and nurses gave her some basic tips to help her with these side effects and lifestyle changes she would need to make. I will share these tips in the following chapters.

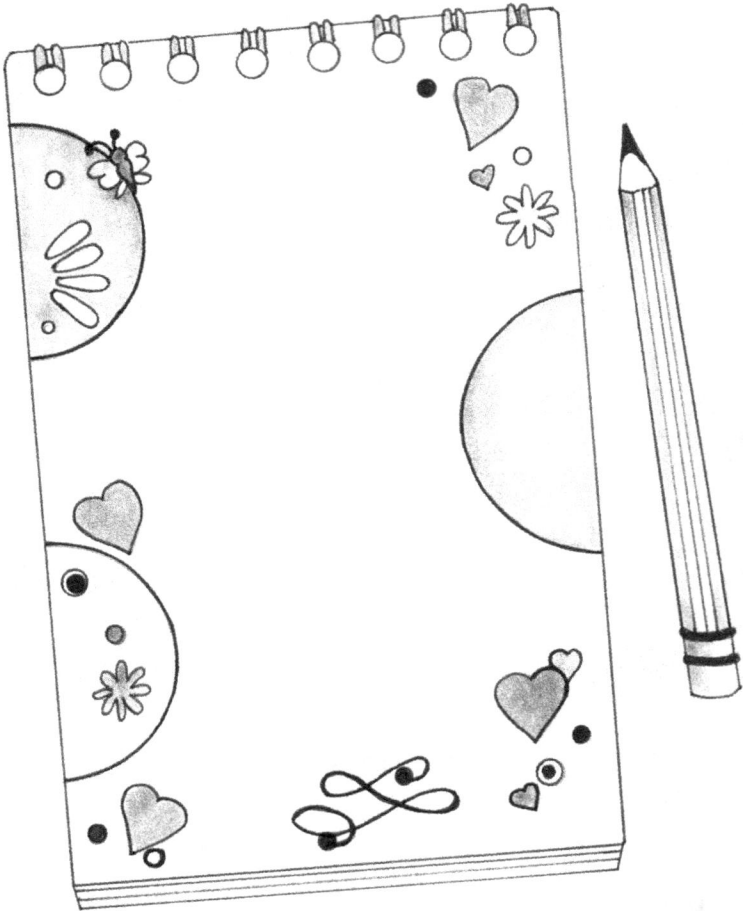

CHAPTER 2

Making changes

My mom was a junk-food junkie! Fast food, candies, cookies, cakes, ice cream . . . she loves it all, let me tell you! When she was pregnant with me, her friends teased her by saying that I was going to come out looking like a Twinkie!

However, mom jumped right in and made the changes she needed to make, per her doctor's instructions. From the day she was diagnosed, she began to change her eating habits. She told me she felt that if she had taken care of the inside of her body, maybe she would not have cancer. She wasn't going to make that mistake anymore.

So, not only she, but we began to change what we were feeding our bodies. Along the way, we learned so much.

For example, chemicals and sugar-filled foods may increase our risk of cancer. Friends and family gave my mom so many books, computer links, and recipes to read. But between her doctor appointments, her business, and her books (she's been a published author for years), and of course, taking care of me and the house, she was always too tired to read. It seemed like a vicious circle: need to read but can't because the cancer made her so exhausted.

So, we talked about it and created a "cheat sheet" to help us stay on track. We even talked about going vegan, but we decided that as healthy as it can be, it was not a diet we would be able to commit to.

We really do try to follow the new rules, but honestly, it is so easy to go back to our old habits, and we often have to remind one another of our healthy-eating goals.

CHAPTER 3

Tricks and tips

When mom was telling me about side effects she may have, the one that really stood out for me was that her food would taste funny, like metal. But there is a way to combat that problem. The trick? Use plastic utensils! How easy is that? And that's exactly what Mom did.

Feeling exhausted is another side effect, not just of the treatment but also of the cancer itself. The trick? It's a pretty obvious remedy, but not so easy for my mom, who is constantly on the go. SLEEP! Even healthy bodies need rest. People with cancer, undergoing chemotherapy, need lots of rest to have energy for the next day and keep their brains sharp. Mom did her best to make sure she was rested so she could handle all the many parts of her life that are so important to our family.

My mom was also reminded to drink lots of water to stay hydrated and allow her body to work at maximum capacity. Remember, our body is made up of 70% water. We need it to survive. Not from a plastic bottle, though. The plastic has chemicals in it.

Filtered water is better, but cancer patients should really drink (natural) alkaline water. Alkaline water is great for anyone, kids included! It is loaded with natural minerals. Alkaline is the opposite of acidic and can help balance our body's pH levels. I read that alkaline water helps improve blood circulation. Foods which contain high alkaline levels are also really good for us – like avocados (which I am not really a fan of), asparagus (I love how my mom makes them), apples (I love them with some cinnamon), almonds (a great snack), broccoli (no comment), cucumbers, green beans, spinach (I try. I really do. My favorite way to eat it is in Greek spinach pie). Have you ever tried butternut squash spaghetti? YUM! And believe it or not, watermelon! How fun is that? These foods not only are high in alkaline but are nutritious. They may contain protein, vitamins and/or minerals. Each benefits our bodies in so many different ways and are known for their antioxidant and anti-inflammatory properties.

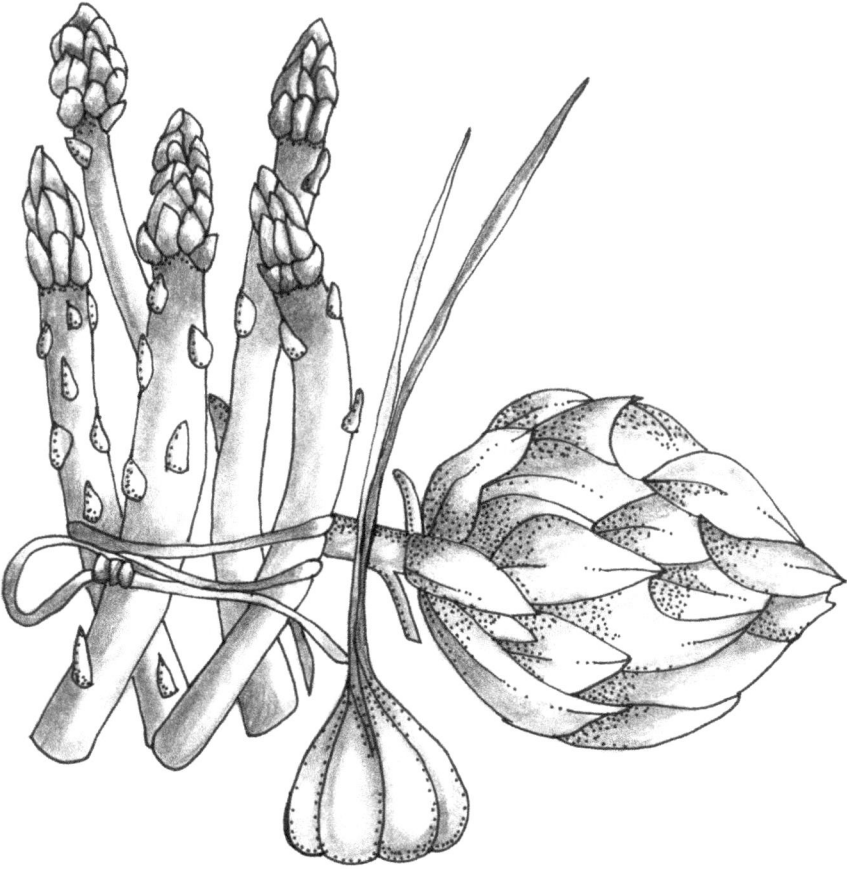

CHAPTER 4

A healthier us

You're never too young to focus on what you feed your body. That is one thing I've learned and taken to heart. My mom and I now work together to ensure we are giving our bodies and minds the best chance to thrive. It's a team effort, for sure. I help whenever and however I can. I like to think that I've made a difference by being a partner in her recovery.

As I mentioned earlier, the number one rule for cancer patients is to stop eating sugar! Sugar feeds the cancer, causing it to grow.

When my mom and I go shopping, we pay attention to the ingredient labels. The first thing we look at is the amount of sugar. If it reads "0 grams," it's perfect. I must confess, there are some things we just have to have! My mom and I both love our sweets, so it's a bit difficult at times. Eating lots of fruits fixes the sweet tooth right up! I never really wanted to eat fruits and veggies before, but one by one, I am learning to like them.

Since carbohydrates turn to sugar, we also look at

the carbohydrate content in our foods. We also search for foods that have as few ingredients as possible. That means the food is more natural. I've seen some foods with twenty different ingredients, most of which I can't even pronounce. Those are most likely chemicals, and not healthy for our bodies. Avoid!

There is a big difference between "added sugar" and "natural sugars," such as fruit sugars. Keep your eyes open in that regard as well.

"Organic" is a word we had been familiar with, but never really paid much attention to before mom's diagnosis. It refers to the way farmers grow and process our foods, including meats, dairy, fruits, vegetables, and grains. "Organic" basically means that farmers do not use harmful chemical fertilizers or pesticides. If those things kill bugs, just think what they can do to our bodies! No thanks!

We've talked about nourishing our inner bodies, so now let's talk about nourishing our outer bodies!

CHAPTER 5

Skincare

Remember, what we put onto our skin goes into our bodies. Just like the ingredient labels on our foods, we must look at the labels on cosmetics. Shampoos and all those yummy-smelling soaps, lotions, and gels have loads of chemicals, which our bodies absorb through our pores. That includes deodorant!

Never fear, though. Mom and I have learned there are so many options that are healthier for our skin and bodies. You want to look for products that contain no aluminum, parabems, flouride, or alcohol. Seek and you shall find!

We use natural oils for a variety of things—to shave, to moisturize our skin, to condition our hair, as a bug repellant, a decongestant, to calm itching from mosquito bites, and Mom uses one to help her high blood pressure . . . and they smell so delicious! Well, most of them do.

CHAPTER 6

Super foods in review

Mom and I have discovered some excellent foods in particular which help cancer patients. (But always check with the doctor first!)

The G-BOMBS: Greens, Beans, Onions, Mushrooms, Berries, Seeds.

Apple cider vinegar is great on salads and helps with so many things, like weight loss. It lowers cholesterol and reduces allergy symptoms.

Baking soda is high in alkaline. Mix it with water and drink up!

Budwig Protocol Diet – It's a combination of cottage cheese, flax oil, and grounded flax seeds. It may not sound very appetizing, but add fruits and nuts to the top, and it tastes like an amazing oatmeal!

Flax seeds have been around for thousands of years. They add a really nice crunch to a bland salad and are known to help prevent diabetes, cholesterol, and cancer, just to name a few.

Water with a whole lemon every morning does amazing things for the digestive system!

Lots of fruits and veggies, raw or cooked. Some

fruits and veggies lose a lot of their vitamins and nutrients when heated, while others hold on to them. Pineapples, mangos, and papayas contain very important digestive enzymes. The extract oil of fruits and vegetables provide a variety of healing elements.

Vitamins and supplements are a must, under your doctor's guidance. My mom loves her turmeric curcumin, which acts as anti-inflammatory. When the inflammation goes down, she has less pain.

AVOID: sugar, dairy, gluten, animal protein.

CHAPTER 7

The air that we breathe

If you are near someone who is smoking, ask the adult you are with if you can move somewhere else. Some adults who smoke in the car with their kids in the back seat think that it is okay if they open the windows. Think about it . . . the smoke just blows to the back! Considering that my dad was a heavy smoker, I often find myself looking up information about the effects of smoking. Second-hand smoke is even more dangerous than what smokers are actually breathing into their lungs. The Centers for Disease Control and Prevention (CDC) has very informative and easy to understand statistics on their website. One bullet point which really hit a nerve read: "Tobacco smoke contains more than 7,000 chemicals, including hundreds that are toxic and about 70 that can cause cancer."

The new fad is vaping. Everyone seems to think vaping is so much safer and an alternative to cigarettes. NOT! Have you ever heard of "popcorn lungs"? In short, the e-cigarette's fluid contains the chemical diacetyl, which damages your lungs airways, causing you to cough and making you feel short of breath. Take a look at the American Lung Association's website to learn more about this!

House cleaners can have lots of chemicals in them, even the ones which smell nice, but they are not good for our bodies, inside or out. Unscented is the way to go! White vinegar is a great alternative to keep things environmentally safe!

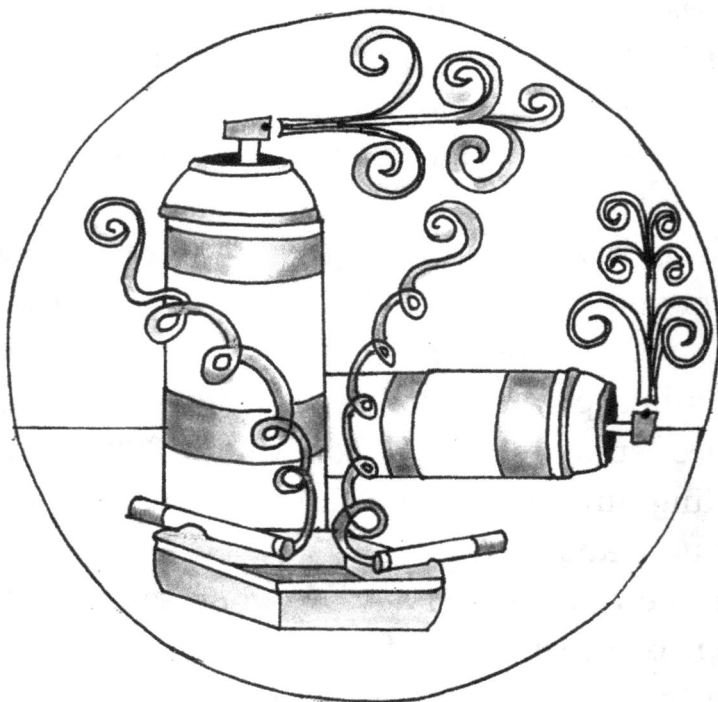

Glossary*

ALKALINE: of, relating to, containing, or having the properties of an alkali or alkali metal; especially, of a solution; having a pH of more than 7.

ENVIRONMENTALLY SAFE: not environmentally harmful, not having a bad effect on the natural world.

EXTRACTS: a product (such as an essence or concentrate) prepared by extracting; especially, a solution (as in alcohol) of essential constituents of a complex material (such as meat or an aromatic plant).

GLUTEN: a gluey protein substance especially of wheat flour that causes dough to be sticky.

HERBS: 1: a seed-producing plant that does not develop persistent woody tissue but dies down at the end of a growing season. 2: a plant or plant part valued for its medicinal, savory, or aromatic qualities.

ORGANIC: of, relating to, yielding, or involving the use of food produced with the use of feed or fertilizer of plant or animal origin without employment of chemically formulated fertilizers, growth stimulants, antibiotics, or pesticides.

PARABEN: either of two antifungal agents used as preservatives in foods and pharmaceuticals: a: METHYLPARABEN b: PRO-PYLPARABEN.

PURE: (1): unmixed with any other matter (2): free from dust, dirt, or taint.

RAW: (1): being in or nearly in the natural state, not processed or purified.

UNSCENTED: having no scent, not scented.

VEGAN: a strict vegetarian who consumes no food (such as meat, eggs, or dairy products) that comes from animals.

---

* Merriam-Webster

Katerina Lecourezos
(Daughter)

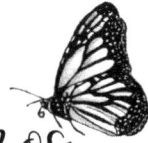

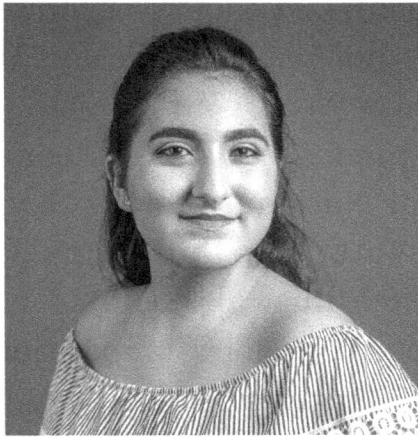

Though Katerina is always proud to share that she was born in Manhattan, she spent her younger years in Queens. After the passing of her dad, she and her mom moved to the hometown of her grandparents, Tarpon Springs, Florida.

At just eleven years old, she was already planning her future, which included attending UCLA to study being a director or cinematographer. The acting/film industry has been her passion ever since. At age fourteen, she auditioned for and was accepted to attend Pinellas County Center for the Arts at Gibbs High School, where she currently attends as a freshman.

During her years at Tarpon Middle School, she was in their Women's Chamber Chorus, elected vice president of the Student Council, was historian for Future Business Leaders of America, and was inducted into the National Junior Honor Society. Additionally, as a World War II history buff, her individual performance on Pearl Harbor earned its way to state level for National History Day.

Katerina has attended the Tampa Bay Performing Arts Academy (for musical theater) for the past seven years and has been on their Competition Team for the past two years. This year, she played Ms. Hannigan in *Annie* and won an award for Excellence in Voice.

She has trained for voice and drama at Ruth Eckerd Hall-Marcia P. Hoffman School of the Arts and at Straz Center, Patel Conservatory for voice and theater. The St. Pete Opera accepted her to perform in their Christmas performance, *Seasonal Sparkle*. Katerina is also a member of the choir and Byzantine choir at her church, where she has also performed as a soloist. She is fluent in Greek and performs with the Omospondia Greek Theater Group. Katerina is also a performer with the Levendia Greek Folk Dance Troupe and is on their competition team this year.

Katerina participated in Industry Network's showcase in Los Angeles, where she came in "top 10" (of 500 talents) for her voice-over and improv, auditioned for agents, and ultimately became agent-represented. She has since modeled and acted in feature and short films, a TV movie, and a web series. Katerina is a member of Women in Film and Television, and of the Tampa Bay Film Society.

She is very involved in her community and volunteers with a number of organizations and events.

(Photo credit: Lekkas Photography)

Demetra Tsavaris-Lecourezos
(Mom)

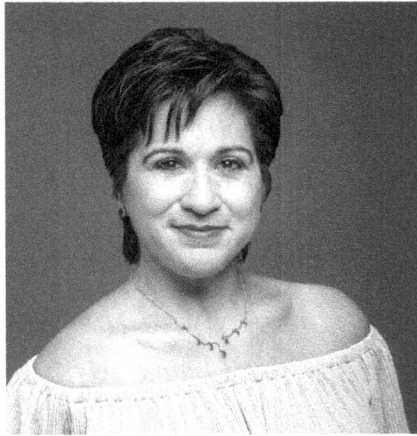

Over the past decade, Demetra has served as caretaker to both her late mother and late-husband; mother to Katerina; "MOMager;" business owner; designer; cancer patient; and renowned author.

All of Demetra's previous books in her Young World Travelers "reference library" have focused on world travel for kids in the form of "EDU-TAINMENT." Demetra never allowed her bout with cancer to interfere with living, writing, and raising Katerina. *Cancer in My Family* was a way to bond with Katerina, to help educate her, and to provide an easy reference guide to better health from the perspective of Katerina's experiences.

Demetra is a member of the Society of Children's Book Writers and Illustrators and a 5-Star recipient from Readers' Favorite.

Her books include:

Young World Travelers
and the Magical Crystal Globe

Ready, Set, OPA!

Letters from Around the World:
Learning the Greek Alphabet

To request an author appearance by Demetra for book signings, storytelling, and author talks, email ywtbooks@gmail.com.

(Photo credit: Lekkas Photography)

Leslie Cronkhite Armstrong

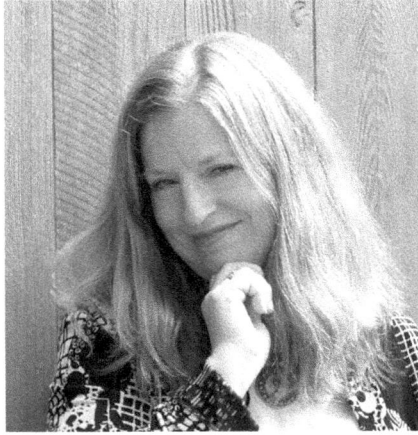

Leslie Cronkhite Armstrong works every day to discover visually what lives in her imagination. Some days are more rewarding than others and being "stuck" occasionally seems to be a part of the process! "The key is to just keep coming to work each day. When things are going well, I am filled with a great sense of wonder and purpose," she says.

Leslie has been teaching, illustrating and designing art curriculum for over 30 years. She holds bachelor's and master's degrees in fine arts and education. Leslie also spent academic time studying art abroad.

Leslie is a member of the Society of Children's

Book Writers and Illustrators and is recognized by Who's Who in American Education.

She has found success as an author, too, with her children's book, *Buster the Dumpster Pony*, based on a true story.

(Photo credit: Joanne Montzingo)

www.ingramcontent.com/pod-product-compliance
Lightning Source LLC
Chambersburg PA
CBHW071942260326
41914CB00004B/728